The Super Easy KETO Chaffle Cooking Guide

Simple And Keto-friendly Chaffle Recipes For Beginners

Lily Sherman

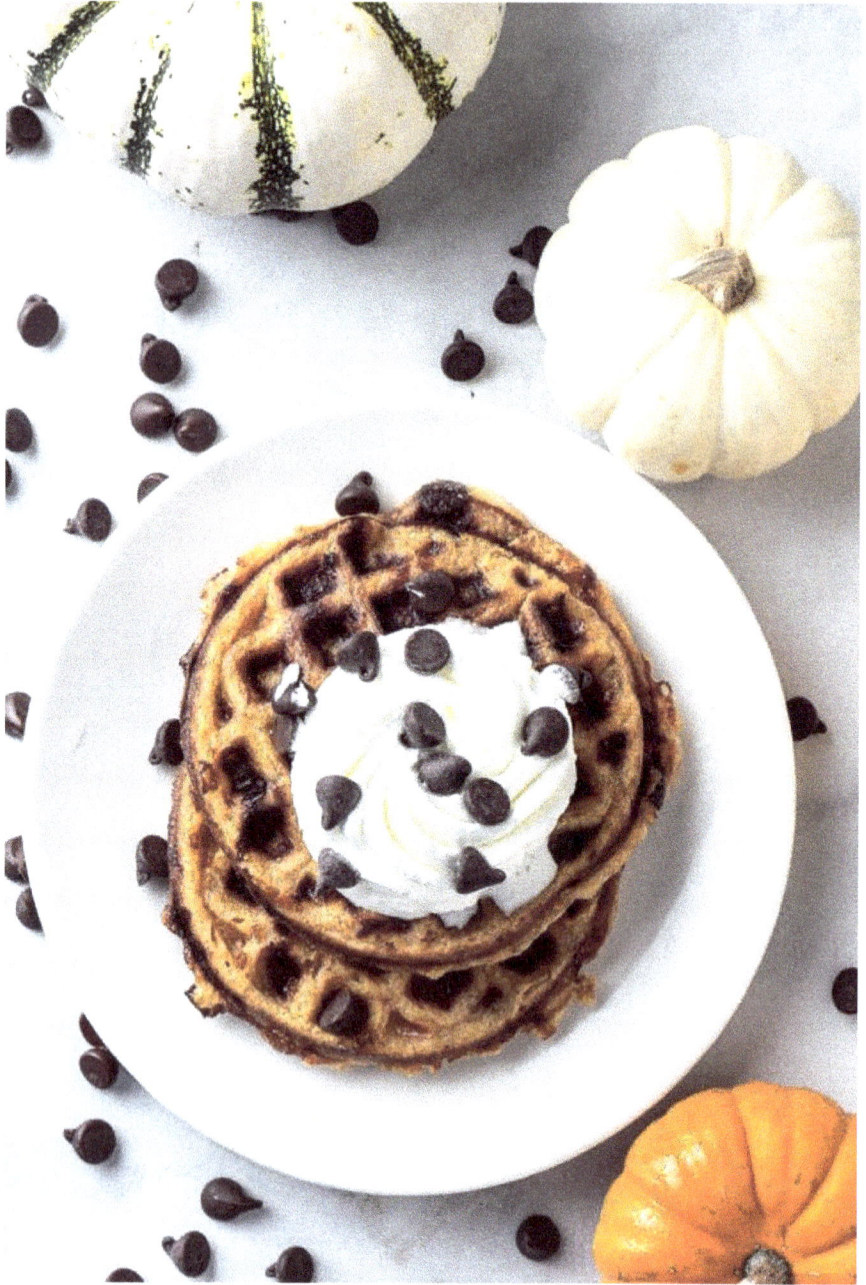

Table of contents

Chicken Bacon Ranch Chaffle

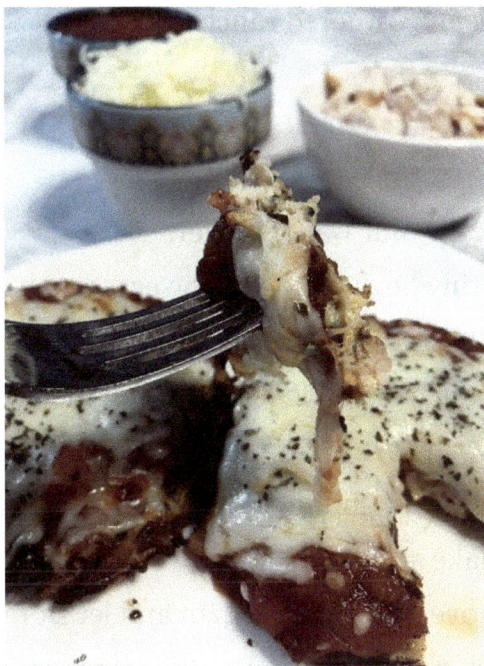

Preparation: 3 minutes

Cooking: 8 minutes

Servings: 2

Ingredients

- 1 egg
- 1/3 cup of cooked chicken diced

- 1 piece bacon cooked and crumbled
- 1/3 cup of shredded cheddar jack cheese
- 1 teaspn powdered ranch dressing

Directions

1. Heat up your waffle maker.
2. In a tiny bowl, mix now the egg, ranch dressing, and Monterey Jack Cheese.
3. Add the bacon and chicken and mix well.
4. Add half of the batter into your waffle maker and cook for 3-4 minutes. Then cook the rest of the batter to make a second chaffle.
5. Remove now from the pan and let sit for 2 minutes.
6. Dip in ranch dressing, sour cream, or enjoy alone.

Chicken Jalapeño Chaffles

Cooking: 14 Minutes

Servings: 2

Ingredients

- 1/8 cup finely grated Parmesan cheese
- ¼ cup finely grated cheddar cheese
- 1 egg, beaten
- ½ cup cooked chicken breasts, diced
- 1 tiny jalapeño pepper, deseeded and minced
- 1/8 tsp garlic powder
- 1/8 tsp onion powder
- 1 tsp cream cheese, softened

Directions

1. Preheat now the waffle iron.
2. In a bowl, mix all the ingredients until adequately combined.
3. Open the iron and add half of the mixture. Close and cook until crispy, 7 minutes.
4. Transfer the chaffle to a plate and make a second chaffle in the same manner.

5. Allow cooling and serve afterward.

Nutrition:

Calories 201, Fats 11.49g, Carbs 3.7, Net Carbs 3.36g, Protein 20.11g

Italian Sausage Chaffles

Preparation: 10 minutes

Cooking: 8 Minutes

Servings: 2

Ingredients

- 1 egg, beaten
- 1 cup cheddar cheese, shredded
- ¼ cup Parmesan cheese, grated
- 1 lb. Italian sausage, crumbled
- 2 teaspns baking powder
- 1 cup almond flour

Directions

- Preheat now your waffle maker.
- Mix all the ingredients in a bowl.
- Pour half of the mixture into your waffle maker.
- Cover and cooking for minutes.
- Transfer to a plate.
- Let cool to make it crispy.

- Do the same steps to make the next chaffle.

Nutrition:

Carbohydrates: 1 g, Fats: 62 g, Proteins: 28 g, Calories: 680

Savory Gruyere & Chives Chaffles

Preparation: 20 minutes

Cooking: 14 Minutes

Servings: 2

Ingredients

- 2 eggs, beaten
- 1 cup finely grated Gruyere cheese
- 2 tbsp. finely grated cheddar cheese
- 1/8 tsp. freshly ground black pepper
- 3 tbsp. minced fresh chives + more for garnishing
- 2 sunshine fried eggs for topping

Directions

1. Preheat now the waffle iron.
2. In a bowl, mix now the eggs, cheeses, black pepper, and chives.
3. Open the iron and pour in half of the mixture.
4. Close the iron and cooking until brown and crispy, 7 minutes.
5. Remove now the chaffle onto a plate and set aside.

6. Make another chaffle using the remaining mixture.

7. Top each chaffle with one fried egg each, garnish with the chives and serve.

Nutrition:

Calories: 402, Total Fat: 30g, Protein: 30g, Total Carbs: 3g, Fiber: 1g, Net Carbs: 2g

Swiss Bacon Chaffle

Preparation: 10 minutes

Cooking: 8 Minutes

Servings: 2

Ingredients

- 1 egg
- ½ cup Swiss cheese
- 2 tbsps cooked crumbled bacon

Directions:

1. Preheat now your waffle maker.
2. Beat the egg in a bowl.
3. Stir in the cheese and bacon.
4. Pour half of the mixture into the device.
5. Close and cooking for 4 minutes.
6. Cooking the second chaffle using the same steps.

Nutrition:

Calories: 317, Total Fat: 18g, Protein: 38g, Total Carbs: 0g, Fiber: 0g, Net Carbs: 0g

Healthy Multigrain Chia Chaffles

Preparation: 15 mins

Cooking: 20 mins

Servings: 8

Ingredients

- 1 3/4 cups almond
- 1 1/4 cups whole
- milk
- wheat flour
- 1/2 cup
- 1/2 cup rolled oats
- unsweetened
- 1/4 cup flax seed
- applesauce
- meal
- 1 egg
- 4 tsp baking powder
- 2 tsp chia seeds
- 2 tsp white sugar
- 1 tsp vanilla extract

- 1/4 tsp salt

Directions

1. Preheat now a Chaffle iron shower within with cooking splash.
2. Whisk almond milk, fruit purée, egg, chia seeds, and vanilla concentrate together in a bowl; let sit until chia seeds begin to thicken the blend, around 2 minutes.
3. Whisk flour, oats, flaxseed supper, preparing powder, sugar, and salt into almond milk blend until the batter is smooth.
4. Scoop 1/2 cup batter into the Preheat Chaffle iron and cook until fresh and brilliant, around 5 minutes for each Chaffle. Rehash with the rest of the batter.

Hot Ham Chaffle

Cooking: 4 Minutes

Servings: 2

Ingredients

- 1/2 cup mozzarella cheese, shredded
- 1 egg
- 1/4 cup ham, chopped
- 1/4 tsp salt
- 2 tbsp mayonnaise
- 1 tsp Dijon mustard

Directions

1. Preheat now your waffle iron.
2. In the meantime, add the egg in a tiny mixing bowl and whisk.
3. Add in the ham, cheese, combine.
4. Scoop half the mixture using a spoon and pour into the hot waffle iron.
5. Close and cook for 4 minutes.
6. Remove now the waffle and place on a large plate. Repeat the process with the remaining batter.

7. In a separate tiny bowl, add the mayo and mustard. Mix well until smooth.
8. Slice the waffles in quarters and use the mayo mixture as the dip.

Nutrition:

Calories: 110 Kcal; Fats: 12 g ; Carbs: 6 g ; Protein: 12 g

Vegan Chaffle

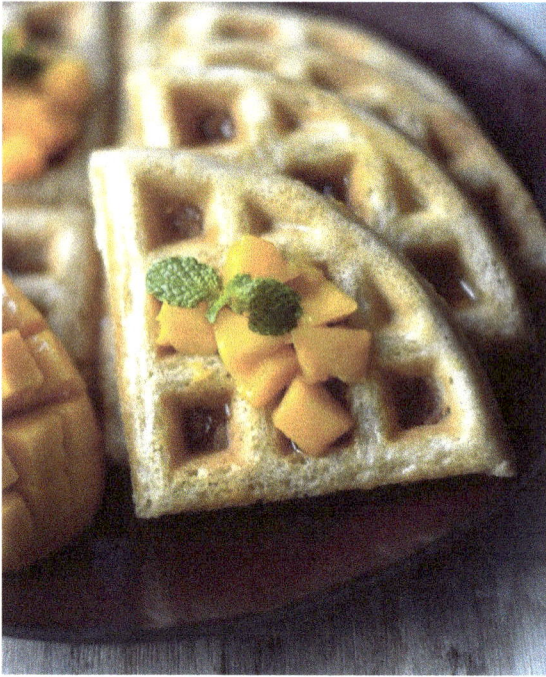

Cooking: 25 Minutes

Servings: 1

Ingredients

- 1 Tbsp flaxseed meal
- 2 1/2 Tbsp water
- 1/4 cup low carb vegan cheese
- 2 Tbsp coconut flour

- 1 Tbsp low carb vegan cream cheese, softened
- Pinch of salt

Directions

1. Turn on waffle maker to heat and oil it, with cooking spray.
2. Mix flaxseed and water in a bowl. Leave for 5 min, until thickened and gooey.
3. whisk remaining Ingredients for Chaffle.
4. Pour one half of the batter into the center of your waffle maker. Close and cook for 3 - 5 minutes.
5. Remove now chaffle and serve.

Nutrition:

Carbs: 3 3 g; Fat: 2 5 g; protein: 25 g; Calories:450

Zucchini Nut Bread Chaffle

Preparation: 20 minutes

Servings: 2

Ingredients

- 1 cup shredded zucchini approximately 1 tiny zucchini
- 1 egg
- 1/2 teaspn cinnamon
- 1 Tbsp plus 1 tsp erythritol blend such as Swerve, Pyure or Lakanto
- Dash ground nutmeg
- 2 tsp Melt butter
- 1 ounce of softened cream cheese
- 2 tsp coconut flour
- 1/2 tsp baking powder
- 3 tbsps chopped walnuts or pecans

Frosting:

- 2 ounce ofs cream cheese at room temperature
- 2 Tbsp butter at room temperature
- 1/4 tsp cinnamon

- 2 Tbsp caramel sugar-free syrup such as Skinny Girl, OR 1 Tbsp confectioner's sweetener, such as Swerve plus 1/8 tsp caramel extract
- 1 Tbsp chopped walnuts or pecans

Directions

1. Grate zucchini and place in a colander over a plate to drain for 15 minutes. With your hands, squeeze out as much moisture as possible.
2. Preheat now the waffle iron until thoroughly hot.
3. In a bowl, whisk all chaffle Ingredients together until well combined.
4. Spoon a heaping 2 tbsps of batter into waffle iron, close and cook 3-5 min, until done.
5. Remove now to a wire rack. Repeat 3 times.

Frosting:

6. Mix all Ingredients together until smooth and spread over each chaffle.
7. Top with additional chopped nuts.

Easy Turkey Burger with Halloumi Cheese Chaffle

Preparation: 20 minutes

Servings: 2

Ingredients

- 1 lb Ground Turkey raw (no need to precook the turkey)
- 8 oz Halloumi shredded
- 1 zucchini medium, shredded
- 2 tbsp Chives chopped
- 1/2 tsp Salt
- 1/4 tsp Pepper

Directions

1. Add all Ingredients to a bowl and mix thoroughly together.
2. Shape into 8 evenly sized patties
3. Preheat now mini griddle.
4. Cook the patties 5-7 minutes

Halloumi Cheese Chaffle

Preparation: 15 minutes

Servings: 3

Ingredients

- 3 oz Halloumi cheese
- 2 T Pasta sauce optional

Directions

1. Cut Halloumi cheese into 1/2 inch thick slices.
2. Place cheese in the UNHEATED waffle maker.
3. Turn waffle maker on.
4. Let it cook for about 3-6 minutes or until golden brown and to your liking.
5. Let cool on a rack for a few minutes.
6. Add Low Carb marinara or pasta sauce.
7. Serve immediately. Enjoy!

Ham Sandwich Chaffles

Cooking: 8 Minutes

Servings: 2

Ingredients

- 1 organic egg, beaten
- 1/2 cup Monterrey Jack cheese, shredded
- 1 teaspn coconut flour
- Pinch of garlic powder

Filling:

- 2 sugar-free ham slices
- 1 tiny tomato, sliced
- 2 lettuce leaves

Directions

- Preheat now a mini waffle iron and then grease it.

For chaffles:

1. In a bowl, put all Ingredients and with a fork, Mix well until well combined. Place half of the mixture into Preheat waffle iron and cook for about 3-4 minutes.

26

2. Repeat now with the remaining mixture.

3. Serve each chaffle with filling Ingredients.

Nutrition:

Net Carbs 3.7 g, Total Fat 8.7 g, Saturated Fat 3.4 g, Cholesterol 114 mg, Sodium 794 mg, Total Carbs 5.5 g, Fiber: 1.8 g Sugar 1.5 g, Protein 13.9 g

Chicken Sandwich Chaffles

Cooking: 8 minutes

Servings: 2

Ingredients

Chaffles:

- 1 large organic egg, beaten
- 1/2 cup cheddar cheese, shredded
- Pinch of salt and ground black pepper

Filling:

- 1 (6-ounce of) cooked chicken breast, halved
- 2 lettuce leaves
- 1/4 of tiny onion, sliced
- 1 tiny tomato, sliced

Directions

1. Preheat now a mini waffle iron and then grease it.

For chaffles:

2. In a bowl, put all Ingredients and with a fork, Mix well until well combined.

28

3. Place half of the mixture into Preheat nowed waffle iron and cook for about 3-4 minutes.
4. Repeat now with the remaining mixture.
5. Serve each chaffle with filling Ingredients.

Nutritional Values:

Calories 2 Net Carbs 2.5 g Total Fat 14.1 g Saturated Fat 6.8 g Cholesterol 177 mg Sodium 334 mg Total Carbs 3.3 g Fiber 0.8 g Sugar 2 g Protein 28.7 g

Salmon & Cheese Sandwich Chaffles

Cooking: 24 minutes

Servings: 4

Ingredients

Chaffles:

- 2 organic eggs
- 1/2 ounce of butter, Melt
- 1 cup mozzarella cheese, shredded
- 2 tbsps almond flour
- Pinch of salt

Filling:

- 1/2 cup smoked salmon
- 1/3 cup of avocado, peeled, pitted, and sliced
- 2 tbsps feta cheese, crumbled

Directions

- Preheat now a mini waffle iron and then grease it.

For chaffles:

1. In a bowl, put all Ingredients and with a fork, Mix well until combined. Place 1/4 of the mixture into Preheat waffle iron and cook for about 5-6 minutes.
2. Repeat now with the remaining mixture.
3. Serve each chaffle with filling Ingredients.

Strawberry Cream Cheese Sandwich Chaffles

Cooking: 10 minutes

Servings: 2

Ingredients

Chaffles:

- 1 organic egg, beaten
- 1 teaspn organic vanilla extract
- 1 tbspn almond flour
- 1 teaspn organic baking powder
- Pinch of ground cinnamon
- 1 cup mozzarella cheese, shredded

Filling:

- 2 tbsps cream cheese, softened
- 2 tbsps erythritol
- 1/4 teaspn organic vanilla extract
- 2 fresh strawberries, hulled and chopped

Directions

1. Preheat now a mini waffle iron and then grease it.

2. For chaffles, add the egg and vanilla extract and mix well in a bowl.

3. Add the flour, baking powder, cinnamon, and Mix well until well combined.

4. Add the mozzarella cheese and stir to combine.

5. Place half of the mixture into Preheat nowed waffle iron and cook for about 4-minutes.

6. Repeat now with the remaining mixture.

7. Meanwhile, for filling: in a bowl, place all the Ingredients except the strawberry pieces and with a hand mixer, beat until well combined.

8. Serve each chaffle with cream cheese mixture and strawberry pieces.

Nutrition:

Calories 143, Total Fat 10.1 g, Saturated Fat 4.5 g, Cholesterol 100 mg, Sodium 148 mg, Total Carbs 4.1g, Fiber 0.8 g, Sugar 1.2 g, Protein 7.6 g

Egg & Bacon Sandwich Chaffles

Cooking: 20 Minutes

Servings: 4

Ingredients

Chaffles:

- 2 large organic eggs, beaten
- 4 tbsps almond flour
- 1 teaspn organic baking powder
- 1 cup mozzarella cheese, shredded

Filling:

- 4 organic fried eggs
- 4 cooked bacon slices

Directions

1. Preheat now a mini waffle iron and then grease it.
2. In a bowl, put all Ingredients and with a fork, Mix well until well combined. Place half of the mixture into Preheat waffle iron and cook for about 3-5 minutes.
3. Repeat now with the remaining mixture.

4. Repeat now with the remaining mixture.

5. Serve each chaffle with filling Ingredients.

Nutrition:

Calories 197, Total Fat 14.5 g, Saturated Fat 4.1 g, Cholesterol 2 mg, Sodium 224 g, Total Carbs 2.7 g, Fiber 0.8 g, Sugar 0.8 g, Protein 12.9 g

Blueberry Peanut Butter Sandwich Chaffles

Cooking: 10 minutes

Servings: 2

Ingredients

- 1 organic egg, beaten
- 1/2 cup cheddar cheese, shredded

Filling:

- 2 tbsps erythritol
- 1 tbspn butter, softened
- 1 tbspn natural peanut butter
- 2 tbsps cream cheese, softened
- 1/4 teaspn organic vanilla extract
- 2 teaspns fresh blueberries

Directions

1. Preheat now a mini waffle iron and then grease it.
2. For chaffles, add the egg and Cheddar cheese and stir to combine in a tiny bowl.
3. Place half of the mixture into Preheat waffle iron and cook for about 5 minutes.

36

4. Repeat now with the remaining mixture.

5. Meanwhile, for filling: In a bowl, put all Ingredients and Mix well until well combined.

6. Serve each chaffle with peanut butter mixture.

Nutrition:

Calories 143, Net Carbs 3.3 g, Total Fat 10.1 g, Saturated Fat 4.5 g, Cholesterol 100 mg, Sodium 148 mg, Total Carbs 4.1g, Fiber 0.8 g, Sugar 1.2 g, Protein 6 g

Berry Sauce Sandwich Chaffles

Cooking: 8 Minutes

Servings: 2

Ingredients

Filling:

- 3 ounce ofs frozen mixed berries,
- thawed with the juice
- 1 tbspn erythritol
- 1 tbspn water
- 1/4 tbspn fresh lemon juice
- 2 teaspns cream

Chaffles:

- 1 large organic egg, beaten
- 1/2 cup cheddar cheese, shredded
- 2 tbsps almond flour

Directions

1. For berry sauce: in a pan, add the berries, erythritol, water and lemon juice over medium heat and cook

for about 8- min, pressing with the spoon occasionally.

2. Remove now the pan of sauce from heat and set aside to cool before serving.
3. Preheat now a mini waffle iron and then grease it.
4. In a bowl, add the egg, cheddar cheese and almond flour and beat until well combined. Place half of the mixture into Preheat nowed waffle iron and cook for about 3-5 minutes.
5. Repeat now with the remaining mixture.
6. Serve each chaffle with cream and berry sauce.

Nutrition:

Calories 222, Net Carbs 4.9, Total Fat 16 g, Saturated Fat 7.2 g, Cholesterol 123 mg, Sodium 212 mg, Total Carbs 7 g, Fiber 2.3 g, Sugar 3.8 g, Protein 10.5 g

Tomato Sandwich Chaffles

Cooking: 6 Minutes

Servings: 2

Ingredients

Chaffles:

- 1 large organic egg, beaten
- 1/2 cup of jack cheese, shredded
- 1/8 teaspn organic vanilla extract

Filling:

- 1 tiny tomato, sliced
- 2 teaspns fresh basil leaves

Directions

- Preheat now a mini waffle iron and then grease it.

For chaffles:

1. In a tiny bowl, place all the ingredients and stir to combine.
2. Place half of the mixture into Preheat nowed waffle iron and cook for about minutes.
3. Repeat now with the remaining mixture.

4. Serve each chaffle with tomato slices and basil leaves.

Nutrition:

Calories 155, Net Carbs 2.4 g, Total Fat 11.g, Saturated Fat 6.8 g, Sodium 217 mg, Total Carbs 3 g, Fiber 0.6 g, Sugar 1.4 g, Protein 9.6 g

Salmon & Cream Sandwich Chaffles

Cooking: 8 Minutes

Servings: 2

Ingredients

<u>Chaffles:</u>

- 1 organic egg, beaten
- 1/2 cup cheddar cheese, shredded
- 1 tbspn almond flour
- 1 tbspn fresh rosemary, chopped

<u>Filling:</u>

- 1/4 cup smoked salmon
- 1 teaspn fresh dill, chopped
- 2 tbsps cream

Directions

1. Preheat now a mini waffle iron and then grease it.

<u>For chaffles:</u>

2. In a bowl, put all ingredients and with a fork, Mix well until well combined.

3. Place half of the mixture into Preheated waffle iron and cook for about 3-4 minutes.
4. Repeat now with the remaining mixture.
5. Serve each chaffle with filling Ingredients.

Nutrition:

Calories 202, Net Carbs 1.7 g, Total Fat 11g, Saturated Fat 7.5 g, Cholesterol 118 mg, Sodium 345 mg, Total Carbs 2.9 g, Fiber 1.2 g Sugar 0.7 g, Protein 13.2 g

Pork Rind Chaffle

Preparation: 10 minutes

Cooking: 20 minutes

Servings: 4 medium chaffles

Ingredients

- 1.1/3 cup of / 150 grams shredded mozzarella cheese
- 4 eggs, at room temperature
- 2 cups / 475 grams crushed pork rinds
- Sour cream for topping

Directions

1. Take a non-stick waffle iron, plug it in, select the medium or medium-high heat setting and let it Preheat now until ready to use; it could also be indicated with an indicator light changing its color.
2. Meanwhile, prepare the batter, and for this, place pork rind in a food processor and process for 1 minute until mixture resembles grains.
3. Take a large bowl, crack eggs in it, add pork rinds and cheese, and mix with a hand whisk until smooth.

4. Use a spoon to pour one-fourth of the prepared batter into the heated waffle iron in a spiral direction, starting from the edges, then shut the lid and cook for 5 minutes or more until solid and nicely browned; the cooked waffle will look like a cake.
5. When done, transfer chaffles to a plate with a silicone spatula and Repeat now with the remaining batter.
6. Let chaffles stand for some time until crispy, top with a dollop of sour cream and serve.

Cheesy Chicken and Ham Chaffle

Preparation: 5 minutes

Cooking: 12 minutes

Servings: 4 mini chaffles

Ingredients

- 4 tbsps chopped ham
- 1/4 cup / 60 grams diced chicken, cooked
- 1/4 cup / 30 grams shredded Swiss cheese
- 1 egg, at room temperature
- 1/4 cup / 30 grams shredded mozzarella cheese

Directions

1. Take a non-stick mini waffle iron, plug it in, select the medium or medium-high heat setting and let it Preheat until ready to use; it could also be indicated with an indicator light changing its color.

2. Meanwhile, prepare the batter and for this, take a large bowl, crack eggs in it, beat with a hand whisk, then add remaining ingredients and whisk until incorporated.

3. Use a spoon to pour one-fourth of the prepared batter into the heated waffle iron in a spiral direction, starting from the edges, then shut the lid and cook for 4 minutes or more until solid and nicely browned; the cooked waffle will look like a cake.
4. When done, transfer chaffles to a plate with a silicone spatula and Repeat now with the remaining batter.
5. Let chaffles stand for some time until crispy and serve straight away.

Cloud Bread Cheddar Chaffle

Preparation: 10 minutes

Cooking: 20 minutes

Servings: 4

Ingredients

- ¼ cup / 60 grams whey protein powder
- ¼ teaspn salt
- ½ teaspn baking powder
- ¼ cup / 60 grams sour cream
- ½ cup / 55 shredded cheddar cheese
- 3 eggs, at room temperature
- Crispy bacon for topping
- Chopped chives for topping

Directions

1. Take a non-stick waffle iron, plug it in, select the medium or medium-high heat setting and let it Preheat now until ready to use; it could also be indicated with an indicator light changing its color.

2. Meanwhile, prepare the batter and for this, take a large bowl, crack eggs in it, add remaining ingredients except for the toppings and then stir with an electric mixer until smooth.

3. Use a spoon to pour one-fourth of the prepared batter into the heated waffle iron in a spiral direction, starting from the edges, then shut the lid and cook for 5 minutes or more until solid and nicely browned; the cooked waffle will look like a cake.

4. When done, transfer chaffles to a plate with a silicone spatula and Repeat now with the remaining batter.

5. Let chaffles stand for some time until crispy, then top with bacon, sprinkle with chives, and serve straight away.

Brie, Basil and Tomato Chaffle

Preparation: 10 minutes

Cooking: 24 minutes

Servings: 4 mini chaffles

Ingredients

- 4 cherry tomatoes, diced
- 1 teaspn dried basil
- 1 cup / 235 grams Brie cheese cubes, softened
- 2 eggs, at room temperature

Directions

1. Take a non-stick mini waffle iron, plug it in, select the medium or medium-high heat setting and let it Preheat now until ready to use; it could also be indicated with an indicator light changing its color.
2. Meanwhile, prepare the batter and for this, take a large bowl, crack eggs in it, add cheese, tomatoes, and basil and mix with a hand whisk until combined.
3. Use a spoon to pour one-fourth of the prepared batter into the heated waffle iron in a spiral direction,

starting from the edges, then shut the lid and cook for 4 to 6 minutes until solid and nicely browned; the cooked waffle will look like a cake.

4. When done, transfer chaffles to a plate with a silicone spatula and Repeat now with the remaining batter.

5. Let chaffles stand for some time until crispy and serve straight away.

Cheesy Spinach Chaffle

Preparation: 10 minutes

Cooking: 20 minutes

Servings: 4 large chaffles

Ingredients

- 1 cup / 225 grams frozen baby spinach, thawed
- ½ teaspn ground black pepper
- ½ teaspn salt
- ½ teaspn cumin
- 1 cup / 115 grams grated cheddar cheese
- 8 eggs, at room temperature

For the Avocado Sauce:

- 1 medium avocado, pitted, diced
- ¼ teaspn ground black pepper
- 1/3 teaspn salt
- 2 limes, juiced
- 2 tbsps coconut milk, unsweetened

Directions

1. Take a non-stick waffle iron, plug it in, select the medium or medium-high heat setting and let it Preheat now until ready to use; it could also be indicated with an indicator light changing its color.

2. Meanwhile, prepare the batter for the chaffles, and for this, squeeze moisture from the spinach in a fine sieve as much as possible and then chop it.

3. Take a large bowl, add spinach in it along with cheese, cumin, black pepper, salt and eggs, and stir with a hand whisk until smooth.

4. Use a spoon to pour one-fourth of the prepared batter into the heated waffle iron in a spiral direction, starting from the edges, then shut the lid and cook for 5 minutes or more until solid and nicely browned; the cooked waffle will look like a cake.

5. When done, transfer chaffles to a plate with a silicone spatula and Repeat now with the remaining batter.

6. In the meantime, prepare the sauce, and for this, place diced avocado in a blender along with remaining ingredients and process for 1 minute until smooth.

7. Let chaffles stand until crispy, then drizzle with prepared avocado sauce and serve straight away.

Spinach Artichoke Chaffle with Bacon

Preparation: 5 mins

Cooking: 8 mins

Servings: 2

Ingredients

- 4 slices of bacon
- ½ cup chopped spinach
- 1/3 cup of marinated artichoke (chopped)
- 1 egg
- ¼ tsp garlic powder
- ¼ tsp smoked paprika
- 2 tbsp cream cheese (softened)
- 1/3 cup of shredded mozzarella

Directions

1. Heat up a frying pan and add the bacon slices. Sear until both sides of the bacon slices are browned. Use a slotted spoon to transfer the bacon to a paper towel line plate to drain.

2. Once the bacon slices are cool, chop them into bits and set aside.
3. Plug your waffle maker to Preheat now it and spray it with a non-stick cooking spray.
4. In a mixing bowl, combine mozzarella, garlic, paprika, cream cheese and egg. Mix well until the ingredients are well combined.
5. Add the spinach, artichoke and bacon bit. Mix well until they are well incorporated.
6. Pour an appropriate amount of the batter into your waffle maker and spread it to the edges to cover all the holes on your waffle maker.
7. Close your waffle maker and cook 4 minutes or more, according to your waffle maker's settings.
8. After the cooking cycle, use a silicone or plastic utensil to Remove now the chaffle from your waffle maker.
9. Repeat step 6 to 8 until you have cooked all the batter into chaffles.
10. Serve and top with sour cream as desired.

Lobster Chaffle

Preparation: 5 mins

Cooking: 8 mins

Servings: 2

Ingredients

- 1 egg (beaten)
- ½ cup shredded mozzarella cheese
- ¼ tsp garlic powder
- ¼ tsp onion powder
- 1/8 tsp Italian seasoning

Lobster Filling:

- ½ cup lobster tails (defrosted)
- 1 tbsp mayonnaise
- 1 tsp dried basil
- 1 tsp lemon juice
- 1 tbsp chopped green onion

Directions

1. Plug your waffle maker to Preheat and spray it with a non-stick cooking spray.
2. In a mixing bowl, combine the mozzarella, Italian seasoning, garlic and onion powder. Add the egg and Mix well until the ingredients are well combined.
3. Pour an appropriate amount of the batter into your waffle maker and spread out the batter to cover all the holes on your waffle maker.
4. Close your waffle maker and cook for about 4 minutes or according to your waffle maker's settings.
5. After the cooking cycle, use a plastic or silicone utensil to Remove now and transfer the chaffle to a wire rack to cool.
6. Repeat step 3 to 5 until you have cooked all the batter into chaffles.
7. For the filling, put the lobster tail in a mixing bowl and add the mayonnaise, basil and lemon juice. Toss until the ingredients are well combine.
8. Fill the chaffles with the lobster mixture and garnish with chopped green onion.
9. Serve and enjoy.

Ground Beef Chaffles

Cooking: 20 Minutes

Servings: 4

Ingredients

- 1/2 cup cooked grass-fed ground beef
- 3 cooked bacon slices, chopped
- 2 organic eggs
- 1/2 cup Cheddar cheese, shred
- 1/2 cup Mozzarella cheese, shredded
- 2 teaspns steak seasoning

Directions

1. Preheat now a mini waffle iron and then grease it.
2. In a bowl, place all ingredients and Mix well until well combined.
3. Place 1/4 of the mixture into Preheat waffle iron and cook for about 4-5 minutes or until golden brown.
4. Repeat now with the remaining mixture.
5. Serve warm.

Nutrition:

Calories: 211, Carb: 0.g, Fat: 12g, Saturated Fat: 5.7g,
Carbohydrates: 0.5 g, Sugar: 0.2g, Protein:2.1g

Salmon Chaffles

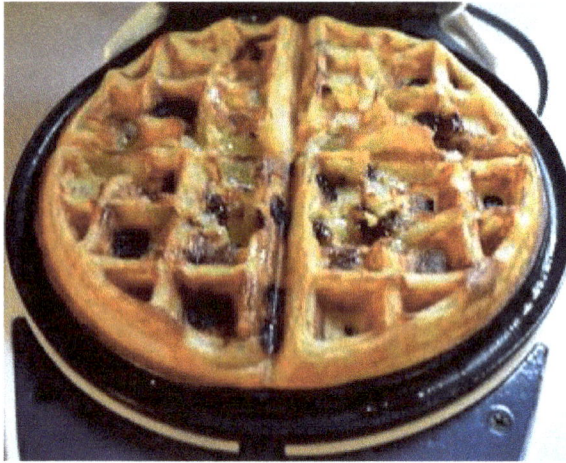

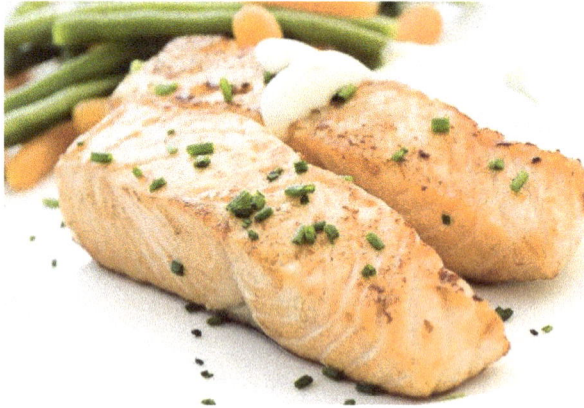

Cooking: 10 Minutes

Servings: 2

Ingredients

- 1 large egg
- 1/2 cup shredded mozzarella
- 1 Tbsp cream cheese
- 2 slices salmon
- 1 Tbsp everything bagel seasoning

Directions

1. Turn on waffle maker to heat and oil it with cooking spray.
2. Beat egg in a bowl, then add 1/2 cup mozzarella.
3. Pour half of the mixture into maker and cook for 4 minutes.
4. Remove now and Repeat now with remaining mixture.
5. Let chaffles cool, then spread cream cheese, sprinkle with seasoning, and top with salmon.

Nutrition:

Carbs: 3 g; Fat: 10 g; Protein: 5 g ;Calories: 201

Chaffle Katsu Sandwich

Cooking: 20 Minutes

Servings: 4

Ingredients

For the chicken:

- 1/4 lb boneless and skinless thigh
- 1/8 tsp salt
- 1/8 tsp black pepper
- 1/2 cup almond flour
- 1 egg
- 3 oz unflavored pork rinds
- 2 cup vegetable oil for deep frying

For the brine:

- 2 cups of water
- 1 Tbsp salt

For the sauce:

- 2 Tbsp sugar-free ketchup
- 1 1/2 Tbsp Worcestershire Sauce
- 1 Tbsp oyster sauce
- 1 tsp swerve/monk fruit

For the chaffle:

- 2 egg
- 1 cup shredded mozzarella cheese

Directions

1. Add brine ingredients in a large mixing bowl.
2. Add chicken and brine for 1 hour.
3. Pat chicken dry with a paper towel. Sprinkle with salt and pepper. Set aside.
4. Mix Ketchup, oyster sauce, Worcestershire sauce, and swerve in a tiny mixing bowl.
5. Pulse pork rinds in a food processor, making fine crumbs.
6. Fill one bowl with flour, a second bowl with beaten eggs, and a third with crushed pork rinds.
7. Dip and coat each thigh in flour, eggs, crushed pork rinds. Transfer on holding a plate.
8. Add oil to cover 1/2 inch of frying pan, Heat to 375 ° F.
9. Once oil is hot, reduce heat to medium and add chicken. Cooking time depends on the chicken thickness.
10. Transfer to a drying rack.

11. Turn on waffle maker to heat and oil it with cooking spray.
12. Beat egg in a tiny bowl.
13. Place 1/8 cup of cheese on waffle maker, then add 1/4 of the egg mixture and top with 1/8 cup of cheese.
14. Cook for 3 -4 minutes.
15. Repeat tor remaining batter.
16. Top chaffles with chicken katsu, 1 Tbsp sauce and another piece of chaffle

Nutrition:

Carbs: 12 g ; Fat: 1g; Protein: 2g ;Calories: 57

Easy Chicken Parmesan Chaffle

Preparation: 15 minutes

Servings: 2

Ingredients

Chaffle:

- 1/2 cup canned chicken breast
- 1/4 cup cheddar cheese
- 1/8 cup parmesan cheese
- 1 egg
- 1 tsp Italian seasoning
- 1/8 tsp garlic powder
- 1 tsp cream cheese room temperature

Topping:

- 2 slices of provolone cheese
- 1 tbs sugar free pizza sauce

Directions

1. Preheat now the mini waffle maker.
2. In a medium-size bowl, add all the ingredients and Mix well until it's fully incorporated.

3. Add a teaspn of shredded cheese to the waffle iron for 30 seconds before adding the mixture. This will create the best crust and make it easier to take this heavy chaffle out of your waffle maker when it's done.
4. Pour half of the mixture in the mini waffle maker and cook it for a minimum of 4 to 5 minutes.
5. Repeat the above steps to cook the second Chicken Parmesan Chaffle.

Nutrition:

Total Fat 21.8g 28%, Cholesterol 134.6mg 45%, Sodium 871mg 38%, Total Carbohydrate 9.2g 3%, Dietary Fiber 2.3g 8%, Sugars 4.7g, Protein 18.5g 37%, Vitamin A 163.1µg 18%

Pork Rind Chaffles

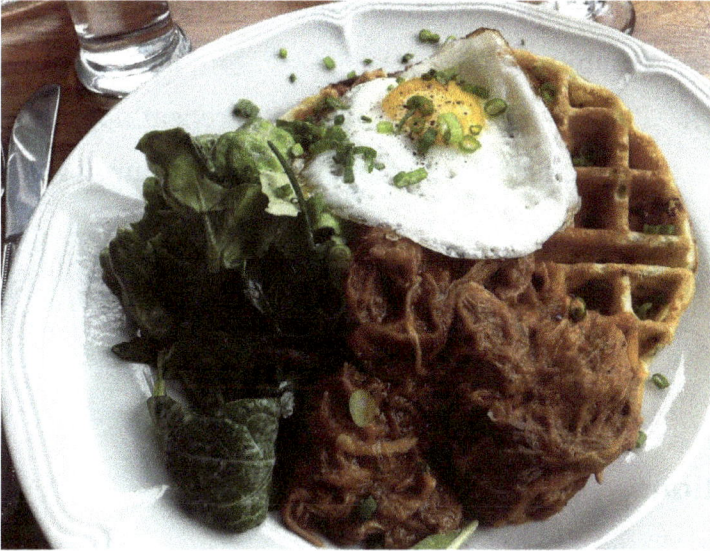

Cooking: 10 Minutes

Servings: 2

Ingredients

- 1 organic egg, beaten
- 1/2 cup ground pork rinds
- 1/ 3 cup Mozzarella cheese, shredded
- Pinch of salt

Directions

1. Preheat now a mini waffle iron and then grease it.
2. In a bowl, place all the ingredients and beat until well combined.
3. Place half of the mixture into Preheat nowed waffle iron and cook for about 5 minutes or until golden brown.
4. Repeat now with the remaining mixture.
5. Serve warm.

Nutrition:

Calories: 91, Net Carb: 0. 3 g, Fat: 5.9 g, Saturated Fat: 2.3 g, Carbohydrates 0.3g, Sugar: 0.2g, Protein 9.2g

Chicken & Ham Chaffles

Cooking: 16 Minutes

Servings: 4

Ingredients

- 1/4 cup grass-fed cooked chicken, chopped
- 1 ounce of sugar-free ham, chopped
- 1 organic egg, beaten
- 1/4 cup Swiss cheese, shredded
- 1/4 cup Mozzarella cheese, shredded

Directions

1. Pre-heat a mini waffle iron and then grease it.
2. In a bowl, place all ingredients and Mix well until well combined.
3. Place 1/4 of the mixture into Preheat waffle iron and cook for about 4 minutes or until golden brown.
4. Repeat now with the remaining mixture.
5. Serve warm.

Nutrition:

Calories: 71, Net Carb: 0.7g, Fat: 4.2g, Saturated Fat: 2g, Carbohydrates: 0.8 g, Dietary Fiber: 0.1g, Sugar: 0.2g, Protein: 7.4g

Bacon & 3-cheese Chaffles

Cooking: 8 Minutes

Servings: 4

Ingredients

- 3 large organic eggs
- 1/2 cup Swiss cheese, grated
- 1/3 cup of Parmesan cheese, grated
- 1/4 cup cream cheese, softened
- 4 tbsps almond flour
- 1 tbspn coconut flour
- 1/2 teaspn onion powder
- 1/2 teaspn garlic powder
- 1/2 teaspn dried basil, crushed
- 1/2 teaspn dried oregano, crushed
- 1/2 teaspn organic baking powder
- Salt and freshly ground black pepper, to taste
- 4 cooked bacon slices, cut in half

Directions

1. Preheat now a waffle iron and then grease it.

2. In a bowl, place all the ingredients excepting for bacon and Mix well until well combined.

3. Place 1/4 of the mixture into Preheat nowed waffle iron.

4. Arrange 2 halved bacon slices over mixture and cook for about 2 minutes or until golden brown.

5. Repeat now with the remaining mixture and bacon slices,

6. Serve warm

Nutrition:

Carb: 3.2g, Fat: 20.1g, Saturated Fat 8g, Carbohydrates: 4.8g, Dietary Fiber: 1.6g, Sugar: 1g, Protein: 13.9g

Spinach Chaffles

Cooking: 20 Minutes

Servings: 4

Ingredients

- 1 large organic egg, beaten
- 1 cup ricotta cheese, crumbled
- 1/2 cup Mozzarella cheese, shredded
- 1/4 cup Parmesan cheese, grated
- 4 ounce ofs frozen spinach, squeezed
- 1 garlic clove, minced
- Salt and freshly ground black pepper, to taste

Directions

1. Preheat now a mini waffle iron and then grease it.
2. In a bowl, place all ingredients and Mix well until well combined.
3. Place 1/4 of the mixture into Preheat waffle iron and cook for about 4-5 minutes or until golden brown.
4. Repeat now with the remaining mixture
5. Serve warm.

Nutrition:

Calories: 139, Net Carb: 4.3 g, Fat: 8.1g, Saturated Fat: 4g, Carbohy- drates: 4.7g, Dietary Fiber: 0.4g, Sugar: 0.4g, Protein: 12.5 g

Chaffles With Prawns, Cauliflower and Zucchini

Cooking: 10 Minutes

Servings: 3

Ingredients

Chaffle:

- 1 large egg
- 1 tbsp. almond flour
- 1 tbsp. full-fat Greek yogurt
- 1/8 tsp baking powder
- 1/4 cup shredded Swiss cheese

Topping:

- 4oz. grilled prawns
- 4 oz. steamed cauliflower mash
- 1/2 zucchini sliced
- 3 lettuce leaves
- 1 tomato, sliced
- 1 tbsp. flax seeds

Directions

1. Make 3 chaffles with the given chaffles Ingredients.
2. For serving, arrange lettuce leaves on each chaffle.
3. Top with zucchini slice, grill prawns, cauliflower mash and a tomato slice.
4. Drizzle flax seeds on top. Serve and enjoy!

Nutrition:

Protein: 45% 71 kcal, Fat: 47% 75 kcal, Carbohydrates: 8% 12 kcal

Buffalo Hummus Beef Chaffles

Cooking: 32 Minutes

Servings: 4

Ingredients

- 2 eggs
- 1 cup + ¼ cup finely grated cheddar cheese, divided
- 2 chopped fresh scallions
- Salt and freshly ground black pepper to taste
- 2 chicken breasts, cooked and diced
- ¼ cup buffalo sauce
- 3 tbsp low-carb hummus
- 2 celery stalks, chopped
- ¼ cup crumbled blue cheese for TOPPING

Directions

1. Preheat now the waffle iron.
2. In a bowl, mix now the eggs, 1 cup of the cheddar cheese, scallions, salt, and black pepper. Open the iron and add a quarter of the mixture.
3. Close and cook until crispy, 7 minutes.

4. Transfer the chaffle to a plate and make 3 more chaffles in the same manner.
5. Preheat now the oven to 400 F and line a baking sheet with parchment paper. Set aside.
6. Cut the chaffles into quarters and arrange on the baking sheet.
7. In a bowl, mix now the chicken with the buffalo sauce, hummus, and celery.
8. Spoon the chicken mixture onto each quarter of chaffles and top with the remaining cheddar cheese.
9. Place the baking sheet in the oven and bake until the cheese Melt nows, 4 minutes.
10. Remove now from the oven and top with the blue cheese. Serve afterward.

Nutrition:

Calories 552, Fats 28.37g, Carbs 6.97g, Net Carbs 6.07g, Protein 59.8g

Mozzarellas & Psyllium Husk Chaffles

Cooking: 8 Minutes

Servings: 2

Ingredients

- ½ cup Mozzarella cheese, shredded
- 1 large organic egg, beaten
- 2 tbsps blanched almond flour
- ½ teaspn Psyllium husk powder
- ¼ teaspn organic baking powder

Directions

1. Preheat now a mini waffle iron and then grease it.
2. In a bowl, place all the ingredients and beat until well combined.
3. Place half of the mixture into Preheat nowed waffle iron and cook for about 4 minutes or until golden brown.
4. Repeat now with the remaining mixture. Serve warm.

Nutrition:

Calories: 101, Net Carb: 1g, Fat: 7.1g, Saturated Fat: 1.8g, Carbohydrates: 2.9g, Dietary Fiber: 1.3g, Sugar: 0.2g, Protein: 6.7g

Chaffle Minutes Sandwich

Preparation: 10 minutes

Cooking: 10 Minutes

Servings: 2

Ingredients

Chaffle:

- 1 large egg
- 1/8 cup almond flour
- 1/2 tsp. garlic powder
- 3/4 tsp. baking powder
- 1/2 cup shredded cheese

Sandwich Filling:

- 2 slices deli ham
- 2 slices tomatoes
- 1 slice cheddar cheese

Directions

1. Grease your square waffle maker and Preheat now it on medium heat.

2. Mix chaffle ingredients in a mixing bowl until well combined.
3. Pour batter into a square waffle and make two chaffles.
4. Once chaffles are cooked, Remove now from the maker.
5. For a sandwich, arrange deli ham, tomato slice and cheddar cheese between two chaffles.
6. Cut sandwich from the center.
7. Serve and enjoy!

Nutrition:

Protein: 29% 70 kcal, Fat: 66% 159 kcal, Carbohydrates: 4% 10 kcal

Beef Zucchini Chaffle

Preparation: 10 minutes

Cooking: 5 minutes

Servings: 2

Ingredients

- Zucchini: 1 (tiny)
- Beef: ½ cup boneless
- Egg: 1
- Shredded mozzarella: half cup
- Pepper: as per your taste
- Salt: as per your taste
- Basil: 1 tsp

Directions

1. Boil beef in water to make it tender
2. Shred it into tiny pieces and set aside
3. Preheat now your waffle iron
4. Grate zucchini finely

5. Add all the ingredients to zucchini in a bowl and mix well
6. Now add the shredded beef
7. Grease your waffle iron lightly
8. Pour the mixture into a full-size waffle maker and spread evenly
9. Cook till it turns crispy
10. Make as many chaffles as your mixture and waffle maker allow
11. Serve crispy and with your favorite keto sauce

Spinach Beef Chaffle

Preparation: 10 minutes

Cooking: 5 minutes

Servings: 2

Ingredients

- Spinach: ½ cup
- Beef: ½ cup boneless
- Egg: 1
- Shredded mozzarella: half cup
- Pepper: as per your taste
- Garlic powder: 1 tbsp
- Salt: as per your taste
- Basil: 1 tsp

Directions

1. Boil beef in water to make it tender
2. Shred it into tiny pieces and set aside
3. Boil spinach in a saucepan for 10 minutes and strain
4. Preheat now your waffle iron

5. Add all the ingredients to boiled spinach in a bowl and mix well
6. Now add the shredded beef
7. Grease your waffle iron lightly
8. Pour the mixture into a full-size waffle maker and spread evenly
9. Cook till it turns crispy
10. Make as many chaffles as your mixture and waffle maker allow
11. Serve crispy and with your favorite keto sauce

Crispy Beef Burger Chaffle

Preparation: 20 minutes

Cooking: 10 minutes

Servings: 2

Ingredients

For the chaffle:

- Egg: 2
- Mozzarella cheese: 1 cup (shredded)
- Butter: 1 tbsp
- Almond flour: 2 tbsp
- Baking powder: ¼ tsp
- Onion powder: a pinch
- Garlic powder: a pinch
- Salt: a pinch

For the beef:

- Ground beef: 1 lb
- Chives: 2 tbsp
- Cheddar cheese: 1 cup
- Salt: ¼ tsp or as per your taste

- Black pepper: ¼ tsp or as per your taste

Directions

1. Mix all the beef ingredient in a bowl
2. Make patties either grill them or fry them
3. Preheat now a mini waffle maker if needed and grease it
4. In a mixing bowl, add all the chaffle ingredients and mix well
5. Pour the mixture to the lower plate of your waffle maker and spread it evenly to cover the plate properly and close the lid
6. Cook for at least 4 minutes to get the desired crunch
7. Remove now the chaffle from the heat and keep aside for around one minute
8. Make as many chaffles as your mixture and waffle maker allow
9. Serve with the beef patties in between two chaffles

Chicken And Chaffle Nachos

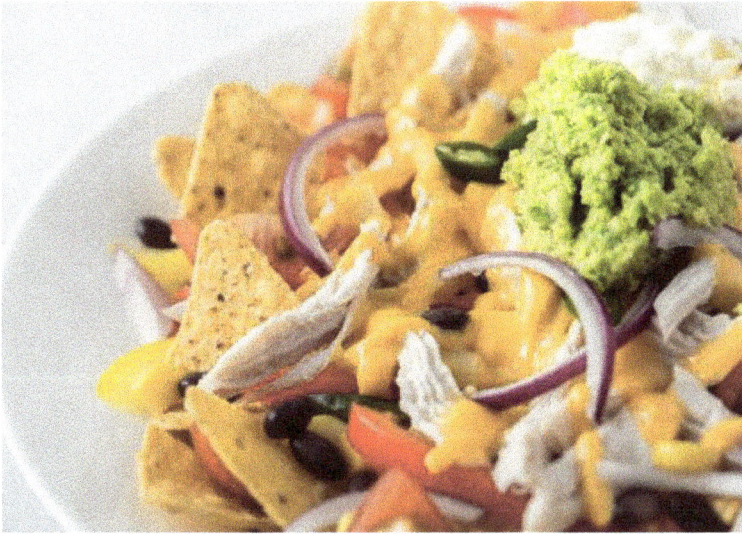

Cooking: 33 Minutes

Servings: 4

Ingredients

For the chaffles:

- 2 eggs, beaten
- 1 cup finely grated Mexican cheese blend

For the chicken-cheese TOPPING:

- 2 tbsp butter
- 1 tbsp almond flour

89

- ¼ cup unsweetened almond milk
- 1 cup finely grated cheddar cheese + more to garnish
- 3 bacon slices, cooked and chopped
- 2 cups cooked and diced chicken breasts
- 2 tbsp hot sauce
- 2 tbsp chopped fresh scallions

Direction

For the chaffles:

1. Preheat now the waffle iron
2. In a bowl, mix now the eggs and Mexican cheese blend.
3. Open the iron and add a quarter of the mixture. Close and cook until crispy, 7 minutes.
4. Transfer the chaffle to a plate and make 3 more chaffles ibn the same manner.
5. Place the chaffles on serving plates and set aside for serving.

For the chicken-cheese tipping:

6. Melt now the butter in a large skillet and mix in the almond flour until brown, 1 minutes.
7. Pour the almond milk and whisk until well combined. Simmer until thickened, 2 minutes.

8. Stir in the cheese to Melt now, 2 minutes and then mix in the bacon, chicken, and hot sauce.

9. Spoon the mixture onto the chaffles and top with some more cheddar cheese.

10. Garnish with the scallions and serve immediately.

Nutrition:

Calories 524, Fats 37.51g, Carbs 3.55g, Net Carbs 3.25g, Protein 41.86g

Bbq Rub Chaffles

Cooking: 20 Minutes

Servings: 4

Ingredients

- 2 organic eggs, beaten
- 1 cup Cheddar cheese, shredded
- 1/2 teaspn BBQ nib
- 1/4 teaspn organic baking powder

Directions

1. Preheat now a mini waffle iron and then grease it.
2. In a bowl, place all ingredients and with a fork, Mix well until well combined.
3. Place 1/4 of the mixture into Preheat nowed waffle iron and cook for about 5 minutes or until golden brown.
4. Repeat now with the remaining mixture.
5. Serve warm.

Nutrition:

Calories: 14, Net Carb: 0.79g, Fat: 11.6g, Saturated Fat: 6.6g, Carbohydrates: 0.79, Dietary Fiber: 0g, Sugar: 0.3g, Protein: 9.8g

Ham Chaffles

Cooking: 16 Minutes

Servings: 4

Ingredients

- 2 large organic eggs (yolks and whites separated)
- 6 tbsps butter, Melt
- 2 scoops unflavored whey protein powder
- 1 teaspn organic baking powder
- Salt, to taste
- 1 ounce of sugar-free ham, chopped finely
- 1 ounce of Cheddar cheese, shredded
- 1/8 teaspn paprika

Directions

1. Preheat now a waffle iron and then grease it.
2. Place egg yolks, butter, protein powder, baking powder and salt, and beat until well combined in a bowl.
3. Add the ham steak pieces, cheese and paprika and stir to combine.

4. Place 2 egg whites and a pinch of salt in another bowl and with an electric hand mixer and beat until stiff peaks form.
5. Gently fold the whipped egg whites into the egg yolk mixture in 2 batches.
6. Place 1/4 of the mixture into Preheat nowed waffle iron and cook for about 3-4 minutes or until golden brown.
7. Repeat now with the remaining mixture.
8. Serve warm.

Nutrition:

Calories: 288, Net Carb: 1.59g, Fat: 22.8g, Saturated Fat: 13.4g, Carbohydrates: 1.79g, Dietary Fiber: 0.2g, Sugar: 0.3g, Protein: 20.3g

Cheddar Jalapeno Chaffle

Cooking: 5 Minutes

Servings: 2

Ingredients

- 2 large eggs
- 1/2 cup shredded mozzarella
- 1/4 cup almond flour
- 1/2 tsp baking powder
- 1/4 cup shredded cheddar cheese
- 2 Tbsp diced jalapenos jarred or canned

For the Toppings:

- 1/2 cooked bacon, chopped
- 2 Tbsp cream cheese
- 1/4 jalapeno slices

Directions

1. Turn on waffle maker to heat and oil it with cooking spray.
2. Mix mozzarella, eggs, baking powder, almond flour, and garlic powder in a bowl.

3. Sprinkle 2 Tbsp cheddar cheese in a thin layer on waffle maker, and 1/2 jalapeno.
4. Spoon half of the egg mixture on top of the cheese and jalapenos.
5. Cook for min, or until done.
6. Repeat for the second chaffle.
7. Top with cream cheese, bacon, and jalapeno slices.

Nutrition:

Carbs: 5 g; Fat: 11g; Protein: 18 g; Calories: 307

Taco Chaffles

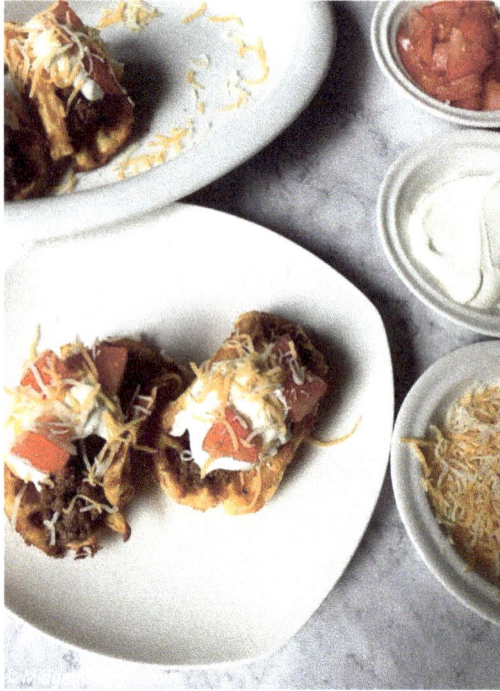

Cooking: 20 Minutes

Servings: 4

Ingredients

- 1 tbspn almond flour
- 1 cup taco blend cheese
- 2 organic eggs

- 1/4 teaspn taco seasoning

Directions

1. Preheat now a mini waffle iron and then grease it.
2. In a bowl, place all ingredients and Mix well until well combined.
3. Place 1/4 of the mixture into Preheat nowed waffle iron and cook for about 4 minutes or until golden brown.
4. Repeat now with the remaining mixture.
5. Serve warm.

Nutrition:

Calories: 71, Net Carb: 0.79g, Fat: 5.4g, Saturated Fat: 2.2g, Carbohydrates: 0.9g, Dietary Fiber: 0.2g, Sugar:0.3g, Protein: 4.59

Spinach & Cauliflower

Cooking: 10 Minutes

Servings: 2

Ingredients

- 1/2 cup frozen chopped spinach, thawed and squeezed
- 1/2 cup cauliflower, chopped finely
- 1/2 cup Cheddar cheese, shredded
- 1/2 cup Mozzarella cheese, shredded
- 1/3 cup of Parmesan cheese, shredded
- 2 organic eggs
- 1 tbspn butter, Melt nowed
- 1 teaspn garlic powder
- 1 teaspn onion powder
- Salt and freshly ground black pepper, to taste

Directions

- Preheat now a waffle iron and then grease it.
- In a bowl, place all ingredients and Mix well until well combined.

- Place half of the mixture into Preheat nowed waffle iron and cook for about 4-5 minutes or until golden brown.
- Repeat now with the remaining mixture.
- Serve warm.

Nutrition:

Calories: 320, Saturated Fat: 14g, Carbohydrates: 59g, Sugar: 1.9g, Protein:20.8g

Zucchini Chaffles With Peanut Butter

Cooking: 5 Minutes

Servings: 2

Ingredients

- 1 cup zucchini grated
- 1 egg beaten
- 1/2 cup shredded parmesan cheese 1/4 cup shredded mozzarella cheese
- 1 tsp dried basil
- 1/2 tsp. salt
- 1/2 tsp. black pepper
- 2 tbsps. peanut butter for TOPPING

Directions

1. Sprinkle salt over zucchini and let it sit for minutes.
2. Squeeze out water from zucchini.
3. Beat egg with zucchini, basil. Salt mozzarella cheese, and pepper.
4. Sprinkle 1/2 of the parmesan cheese over Preheat nowed waffle maker and pour zucchini batter over it.

5. Sprinkle the remaining cheese over it.

6. Close the lid.

7. Cook zucchini chaffles for about 4-8 minutes.

8. Remove now chaffles from the maker and Repeat now with the remaining batter.

9. Serve with peanut butter on top and enjoy!

Nutrition:

Protein: 52% 88 kcal, Fat: 41% 6g kcal, Carbohydrates: 7% 12 kcal

Chicken & jalapeno Chaffles

Cooking: 10 Minutes

Servings: 2

Ingredients

- 1/2 cup grass-fed cooked chicken, chopped
- 1 organic egg, beaten
- 1/4 cup Cheddar cheese, shredded
- 2 tbsps Parmesan cheese, shredded
- 1 teaspn cream cheese, softened
- 1 tiny jalapeno pepper, chopped
- 1/8 teaspn onion powder
- 1/8 teaspn garlic powder

Directions

1. Preheat now a mini waffle iron and then grease it.
2. In a bowl, place all ingredients and Mix well until well combined.
3. Place half of the mixture into Preheat nowed waffle iron and cook for about 4-5 minutes or until golden brown.
4. Repeat now with the remaining mixture.

5. Serve warm.

Nutrition:

Calories: 170, Net Carlo: 0.9g, Fat: 9.9g, Saturated Fat: 5.2g, Carbohy-drates: 0.1g, Oietary Fiber: 2g, Sugar: O. 5g, Protein: 8.6g

Cauliflower & Chives Chaffles

Cooking: 48 Minutes

Servings: 8

Ingredients

- 1/2 cups cauliflower, grated
- 1/2 cup Cheddar cheese, shredded
- 1/2 cup Mozzarella cheese, shredded
- 1/4 cup Parmesan cheese, shredded
- 3 large organic eggs, beaten
- 3 tbsps fresh chives, chopped
- 1/4 teaspn red pepper flakes, crushed
- Salt and freshly ground black pepper, to taste

Directions

1. Preheat now a mini waffle iron and then grease it.
2. In a food processor, Place all the ingredients and pulse until well combined.
3. Divide the mixture into 8 portions.

4. Place 1 portion of the mixture into Preheat nowed waffle iron and cook for about 5-6 minutes or until golden brown.
5. Repeat now with the remaining mixture.
6. Serve warm.

Nutrition:

Net Carb: 1.2g, Fat: 7.3 g, Saturated Fat: 4g, Carbohydrates: 1.7g, Dietary Fiber: 0.5g, Sugar: 0.7g, Protein: 8.8g

Taco Chaffle Shell

Cooking: 8 Minutes

Servings: 1

Ingredients

- 1 egg white
- 1/4 cup shredded Monterey jack cheese
- 1/4 cup shredded sharp cheddar cheese
- 3/4 tsp water
- 1 tsp coconut flour
- 1/4 tsp baking powder
- 1/8 tsp chili powder
- Pinch of salt

Directions

1. Turn on waffle maker to heat and oil it with cooking spray.
2. Mix all components in a bowl.
3. Spoon half of the batter on your waffle maker and cook for 4 minutes.

4. Remove now chaffle and set aside. Repeat for remaining chaffle batter.
5. Turn over a muffin pan and set chaffle between the cups to form a shell. Allow to set for 2-4 minutes.
6. Remove now and serve with your favorite taco.

Nutrition:

Carbs: 4 g, Fat: 19 g, Protein: 18 g, Calories: 258

Pepperoni & Cauliflower Chaffles

Cooking: 16 Minutes

Servings: 4

Ingredients

- 6 turkey pepperoni slices, chopped
- 1/4 cup cauliflower rice
- 1 organic egg, beaten
- 1/4 cup Cheddar cheese, shredded
- 1/4 cup Mozzarella cheese, shredded
- 2 tbsps Parmesan cheese, grated
- 1/2 teaspn Italian seasoning
- 1/4 teaspn onion powder
- 1/4 teaspn garlic powder

Directions

1. Preheat now a mini waffle iron and then grease it.
2. In a bowl, place all ingredients and Mix well until well combined.
3. Place 1/4 of the mixture into Preheat nowed waffle iron and cook for about 4 min, or until golden brown.

4. Repeat now with the remaining mixture

5. Serve warm.

Nutrition:

Calories: 103, Net Carb:0.4g, Fat: 8g, Saturated Fat: 3.2g, Carbohydrates: 0.8g, Dietary Fiber: 0.2g, Sugar: 0.4g

www.ingramcontent.com/pod-product-compliance
Lightning Source LLC
Chambersburg PA
CBHW050747030426
42336CB00012B/1701